Natural Beauty Recipes

Make Makeup In Your Kitchen

Body Peace University

Dr. Felicia Clark

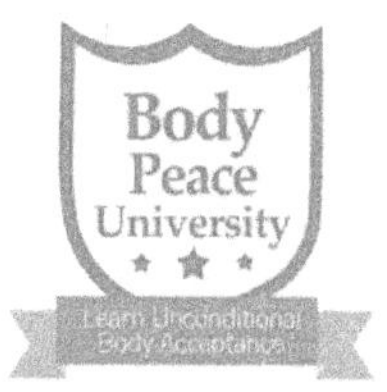

Natural Beauty Recipes: Make Makeup In Your Kitchen

Copyright © 2018 by BodyPeaceUniversity.com Press
Dr. Felicia Clark

ISBN-13:978-1717327451
ISBN-10:1717327451

Dedication

To any woman who has fibroid tumors, fertility challenges, breast cancer, reproductive system cancer or lost her womb due to toxic grooming and beauty products.

Acknowledgement

I wish to acknowledge Cheryl Clark for all of her support, cheerleading, and nudging to make this and several other projects happen for me.

Thank you for believing in me big sis!

This book is used during our live makeup making workshop. It is recommended that you attend a live class and/or register for the online class at:

www.BodyPeaceUniversity.com

Or at

www.DrFeliciaClark.com

Table of Contents

Introduction 7

Your Toolkit 8

Identifying Your Skin Tone 9

Color Pigment and Oils 10

Black Eyeliner/Mascara 11

Face Powder 12

Cream or Liquid Foundation........................... 13

High SPF Cream Foundation 14

Eye Shadow/Blush 15

Lipstick 16

Makeup Remover 17

Night Cream Substitutes 18

Wrinkle Eraser 18

Mask 19

Teeth Whiteners 20

More Tips 21

Introduction

Have you read grooming and beautification product labels and figured out that many of the "health and beauty" products are toxin and beauty products?

You never have to use chemicals whose names you cannot pronounce again – unless you want to. Do you want healthy makeup? I hope so!!

Once you see how SUPER EASY and SUPER AFFORDABLE it is to make your own makeup, you won't want to use toxic expensive products again.

Let's get started!!!

Your Toolkit

Here are great products to keep on hand when you are making makeup. Take a live or online class at bodypeaceuniversity.com to learn hacks to make your dollar stretch further. However, if you make makeup on your own, here is your basic makeup grocery list:

- Activated Charcoal Powder (not the stuff you use to Bar-b-que. STOP IT!)
- Zinc Oxide Powder
- Almond Oil or Argon Oil
- Vitamin E Oil (natural preservative)
- Color Pigment/ Mica Powder
- Coffee Sticks to Stir
- 1-oz disposable plastic cups with lids
- Small Makeup Brushes
- Unrefined honey
- Apple Cider Vinegar

Note: The list is not exhaustive. However, it's enough to keep you in good shape. There are recipes in this book with ingredients not on this list. So, again, the class is highly recommended to best learn what products to use and what can be substituted for the ingredients you have. Join the Making Makeup online class at: www.bodypeaceuniversity.com.

Identifying Your Skin Tone

For the perfect color match of powder and foundation, you will have to play with color combinations.

Everyone will need white and brown. White and brown are used to lighten and darken your makeup mixture. Then look at your skin. You will have a red tint to your skin, a green tint, or a yellow tint. You may need 2 of these tints but rarely all three.

These color combinations make the skin tone of just about everyone's skin tone. You just play with how much of each color you need. And, remember, you will need to lighten or darken your powder and foundation as the seasons change. So, while it's good to write down how much of each color you add, remember that you won't have a standard exact color combination each time.

Color Pigment and Oils

Order mica powder from your favorite vendor in your preferred colors. If you are new and unsure of your colors, <u>Bulk Apothecary</u> has a great sampler pack of pigment colors with all of the colors you will need.

Instead of pigment, you can use food for makeup coloring as follows:

Black – Activated Charcoal Tablets (not the kind you bar-b-que with)

Brown - Cocoa powder, Allspice powder

Brownish-Red – Cinnamon powder

Red – Beetroot powder

Green – Spirulina powder

Pink – break open a hibiscus tea bag in powder form

Yellow – Turmeric powder (it stains so use sparingly)

White – (also used as powder base) arrowroot flour, corn starch, refined coconut powder (ground in coffee grinder)

Oils

Olive, Coconut, or Almond oil can substitute in recipes.

Recommended for eyebrows and lashes – Blackseed oil

Recommended or skin makeup – Argan oil

Black Eyeliner/Mascara

Eyeliner

6 Activated Charcoal Powder Tablets

1-oz disposable cup with lid

Plastic Gloves (optional)

Apply gloves (optional). Break open activated charcoal powder tablets into 1-oz cup. Apply with your favorite makeup brush. Your natural oil will change the consistency of the powder. Cover with lid to store. Note: do not inhale charcoal powder.

Black Eyeliner/Mascara

6 Activated Charcoal Powder Tablets

1-oz disposable cup with lid

1 tsp Blackseed Oil (less or more as desired)

Wooden Coffee Stir Stick

Plastic Gloves (optional)

Apply gloves (optional). Break open activated charcoal powder tablets into 1-oz cup. Add oil (Blackseed oil grows hair but most food liquid oils work). Stir in more oil drops to make thinner. **For Brown** - substitute cocoa powder for charcoal. Apply with your favorite brush. Cover with lid to store. Note: do not inhale charcoal powder.

Face Powder

2 Tbsps of Zinc Oxide Powder

Pinches of brown makeup pigment

A pinch of yellow, red, or green makeup pigment
based on your skin tone

1-oz disposable cup with lid

Mix powder and brown pigment in cup. More brown for darker hues plus a pinch of red, yellow or green until it matches your skin tone. Apply with brush or sponge. Cover and store.

Tips:

Double or triple the recipe. This can be your base for cream foundation, bronzers, and eyeshadow.

Turn into Cream Eyeshadow:

Separate a tsp of the finished powder. Add your favorite colors and 5 (or so) drops of oil to have cream eyeshadow.

Cream or Liquid Foundation

3 Tbsp of Zinc Oxide Powder

A pinch of brown makeup pigment

A pinch of yellow, red, or green makeup pigment
   based on your skin tone

1 tsp Argan Oil

1-oz disposable cup with lid

1-3 tsp water

Wooden Coffee Stir Stick

Stir 2tbsp powder with brown pigment. Add oil. The mixture will become dark brown. Stir in a pinch of red, yellow or green based on your skin tone. It will still be dark. Add 1tsp water and stir. Add more powder to lighten as needed. If too thick, add water. Note: when liquifying, water makes it lighter and oil makes it darker. Apply with a powder brush or makeup sponge. Cover and store.

Tips

Play with this mixture to get your perfect skin tone match and your preferred consistency. More water makes the foundation liquid and lighter in color. More oil makes it creamy and darker. Less liquid makes it a powder/cream foundation. After storing. it will dry out some. Simply scoop dry make up out, wet your sponge and apply semi-dry Makeup with wet sponge. Substitute zinc oxide with coconut powder, flour or cornstarch. The substitution may leave clumps that you dust off with a makeup brush.

High SPF Cream Foundation

1 Tbsp of Zinc Oxide Powder

Pinch of Cocoa Powder

2 Tbsp raw Shea Butter

1 Tbsp raw Cocoa Butter

1 Tbsp of Beeswax

1/8 tsp of Vitamin E oil

3 Tbsp of Almond, Olive or Argan Oil

A pinch of yellow, red, or green makeup pigment

Opt: 1/8th tsp cinnamon powder for bronzing effect

Mix powders, butters and oils until smooth. Stir in cocoa and a pinch of red, yellow or green until it matches your skin tone. Add 1 tsp water and stir. Add more powder to lighten as needed. If too thick, add water. Apply with a powder brush or makeup sponge. Cover and store.

The exact SPF rating is undetermined but it will be around SPF 20.

Eye Shadow/Blush

1/2 tsp arrowroot powder

$\frac{1}{4}$ tsp color powder or pigment

    ---- **(the above is the core powder)**

$\frac{1}{4}$ tsp shea butter (for cream)

Opt: add argan oil drops for heavy application

1 oz plastic cup with lid

Mix powder and color. Add melted butter and/or oil. It should be more dry than oily. Add more arrowroot to lighten eyeshadow color or add more colored power to darken your eyeshadow. Use on eyelids or on cheeks for blush.

Lipstick

1 tsp beeswax pastilles

1 tsp shea butter (sub with cocoa butter)

1 tsp coconut oil

     ---- (the above is lip moisturizer)

1 drop food coloring

$\frac{1}{4}$ tsp bentonite clay (optional for matte finish)

1 drop essential oil for smell (optional)

Melt beeswax, butter and oil in a mini crockpot. Or, put in a shot glass (or other glass jar) and immerse in hot water to melt. DO NOT EXPOSE TO HIGH HEAT.

In a separate shot glass mix clay (optional) and color. Stir color mixture into melted mixture. Let cool.

Optional: Order twist container tubes or small lip gloss tins to store lipstick.

Tip: Play with this recipe until you have your perfect gloss or matte finish and color.

<u>Classic Beauty Tip</u>: make a lipstick the pinkish color of the skin inside of your lip. That's **<u>your</u>** perfect shade.

To color your lipstick: use $\frac{1}{4}$ tsp of your choice

Brown - Cocoa powder

Brownish-Red – Cinnamon powder

Red – Beetroot powder

Pink – open a hibiscus tea bag (powder only)

Makeup Remover

> 1 oz raw honey
>
> 1 oz aloe vera gel
>
> Mix in a jar. Apply with fingers. Wipe off with wash cloth. Note: honey can be used by itself but it is messy.

Option 2

> 1 oz witch hazel
>
> 1 oz water
>
> Mix in a jar. Apply with fingers. Wipe off with cloth.

Make Up Remover Wipes

> 1 Tbsp aloe vera
> 3 tsp witch hazel
> 1 tsp liquid castile soap
> 1 tsp argan oil
> 8-12 drops lavender (optional)
> 1 tsp vitamin E oil (preservative – don't substitute)
> Glass jar with seal
> Cotton rounds
>
> Mix all ingredients in jar. Shake to mix them together. Fill with cotton rounds. Shake until cotton absorbs the mixture. Remove a wet cotton round and use. Reseal jar and keep sealed until ready to use.

Night Cream Substitute

3 tsp argan oil

Wash face with soap and water. Apply argan oil to face as you would night cream. Apply to neck as needed.

Wrinkle Eraser or Prevention

$\frac{1}{2}$ tsp Pure Emu Oil
1 Q-tip

In addition to the argan oil above, apply emu oil in the places where your skin is likely to crack or fold. Apply to mouth corners, side of eyes, brow ridge and neck. If any area is heavily wrinkled or scarred, apply all over the area 3 times per week in place of argan oil.

Mask

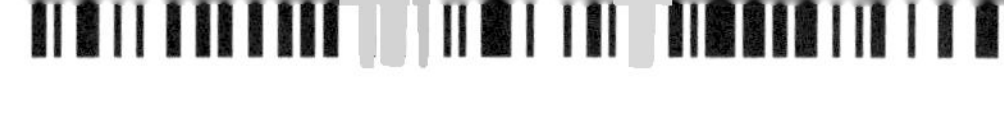

1/8th cup raw unfiltered honey

Paper towels or paper bib

Wash face with soap and water. Apply honey to face and neck. Leave on for as long as you can stand while you work at home. I have left it on up to 5 hours. You will sweat some and the honey will drip. Wear a beat up t-shirt and makeshift paper towel bib to wipe mess. If in a rush, leave on for at least 30 minutes.

Option 2

Fresh Avocado

Wash face with soap and water. Apply the remaining avocado left in the shell after you have scooped the avocado out. (Great to wear this mask while you are making guacamole). Simply snip the avocado skin so it's flat. Rub the skin on your clean face. Leave for 30 minutes to 1 hour. Wash off with a warm wash cloth.

Teeth Whitener

3 tsp baking soda

2 tsp water (can sub with hydrogen peroxide)

Toothbrush

Dip your toothbrush in the mixture and brush teeth as normal.

Option 2

Banana peel

Take a banana peel from a healthy, fresh, yellow banana (not brown). Rub the inside starch part of the banana peel directly on your teeth. It should remove the plaque. Wipe your teeth with a cloth, napkin or brush your teeth as normal.

Option 3

1 oz hydrogen peroxide

Dip your toothbrush in the peroxide and brush as normal.

More Tips

- Add a drop of argan oil to your store bought dry eye shadow and make it a crème eyeliner.

- Wet a q-tip with argan oil. Rub the oil onto your nail cuticles to moisturize them.

- With a q-tip, brush blackseed oil onto your eyelashes and eyebrows to grow them thicker.

- Mix coconut oil with bentonite clay to make a dry paste. Apply it hands, feet, face or back as if you are doing a facial.

- Put raw honey on your hands and feet and wrap them with plastic wrap for an hour. Remove and wash.

Notes:

Record changes you make to recipes.
Record how you blend your favorite colors.

22

Makeup Recipes You Have Discovered:

23

Take a course at: www.BodyPeaceUniversity.com

Sign Up For

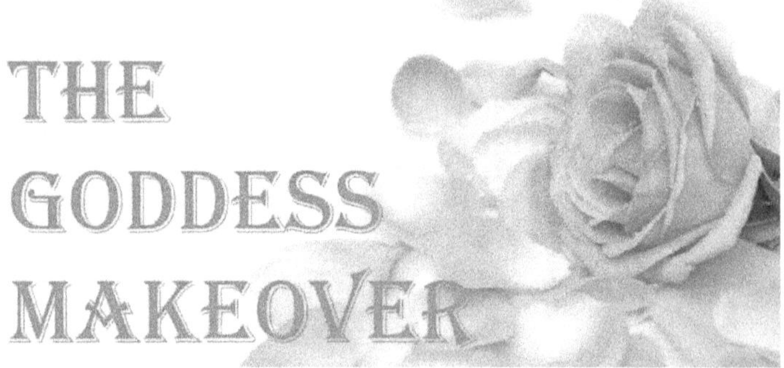

- ✓ Learn the science of beauty
- ✓ Know the 20 classic beauty features for a woman
- ✓ Choose Your 3 lead off features and look like a Goddess in 15 minutes or less!

Join The Sisterhood of Body Peace

- ✓ Receive Body Peace Tips On Your Phone
- ✓ Join an Exclusive Membership Community
- ✓ Interviews From Experts On Body Image
- ✓ Practice Unconditional Body Acceptance

Get your 1-on 1 introductory coaching session with this book's author, Dr. Felicia Clark, to discuss your pathway to body peace. Book here: www.drfeliciaclark.com